Najeh ADAILY
Wafa DAHMANI

CHRONIC LIVER DISEASES

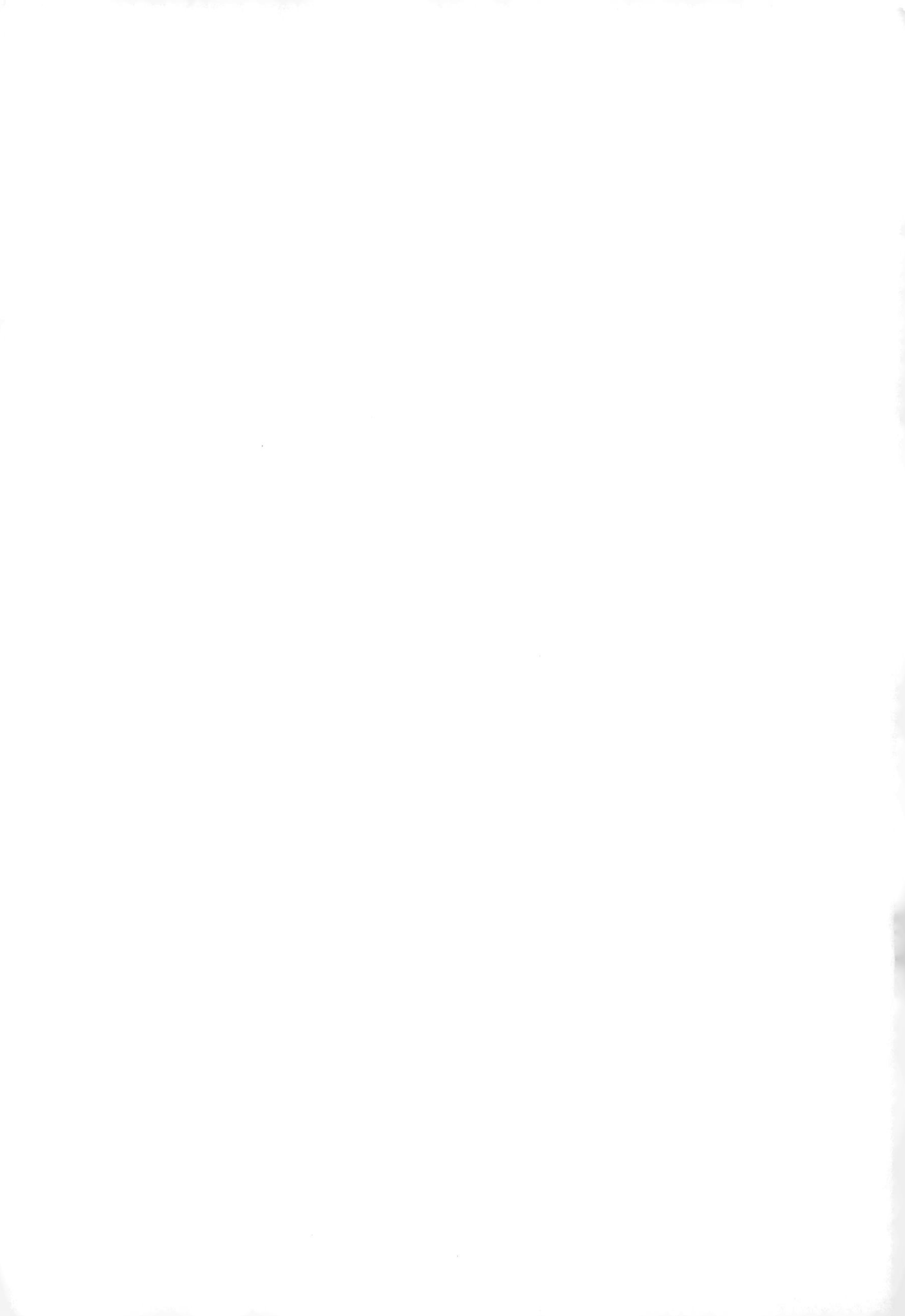

Najeh ADAILY
Wafa DAHMANI

CHRONIC LIVER DISEASES

Evaluation of the perception of chronic liver disease by primary care physicians in Tunisia

ScienciaScripts

Cover image: www.ingimage.com

This book is a translation from the original published under ISBN 978-620-3-45471-0.

Publisher:
Sciencia Scripts
is a trademark of
Dodo Books Indian Ocean Ltd. and OmniScriptum S.R.L publishing group

120 High Road, East Finchley, London, N2 9ED, United Kingdom
Str. Armeneasca 28/1, office 1, Chisinau MD-2012, Republic of Moldova, Europe
Printed at: see last page
ISBN: 978-620-5-89146-9

CHRONIC LIVER DISEASES

EVALUATION OF THE PERCEPTION OF CHRONIC LIVER DISEASE BY PRIMARY CARE PHYSICIANS IN TUNISIA

TABLE OF CONTENTS

INTRODUCTION

Chronic liver diseases, regardless of their cause, can lead to the development of cirrhosis and hepatocellular carcinoma when their evolution is prolonged. They are characterized by persistent inflammation that contributes to their progression to these more severe stages (1,2).

The main causes of chronic liver disease are hepatic steatosis, chronic viral hepatitis B and C and excessive alcohol consumption, which are responsible for more than 90% of cirrhosis cases (2).

Hepatic steatosis has become the **leading cause of chronic liver disease** in the world, due to the global obesity epidemic(3). Its prevalence now exceeds 25% of the world population(4), and 5% of cases progress to advanced liver fibrosis(5).

Hepatitis C virus (HCV) and hepatitis B virus (HBV) are the leading causes of liver cancer and overall mortality worldwide, surpassing malaria and tuberculosis (8).

Excessive alcohol consumption is responsible for 40% of all liver-related deaths (6). According to the results of a recent WHO study

(7), Tunisia occupies the 1st place among Arab countries in terms of alcohol consumption, with an average of **12.92 liters per year and per person;** nevertheless it is difficult to define a threshold of daily consumption that exposes to the risk of developing cirrhosis (6).

Considering the long silent evolution of chronic liver diseases towards advanced stages such as cirrhosis and hepatocellular carcinoma, early detection of all these pathologies represents an important public health issue in Tunisia and in the world.

Indeed, the diagnosis of cirrhosis at the stage of complications is too late because, at that time, the prognosis is very poor with **50% of death at two years** compared to only 5% in the case of compensated cirrhosis (9)· Similarly, **50 to 70%** of primary liver cancers (carcinoma hepatocellular) are diagnosed late and will not be eligible for treatment curative (1).

Thus, general practitioners and family physicians have an essential role to play in screening for chronic liver disease, especially since new and highly effective treatments are now available (3,10,11).

In order to identify early patients who develop advanced liver disease while still asymptomatic, non-invasive fibrosis tests are available (12). They allow the assessment of the degree of hepatic fibrosis in chronic liver disease. The FIB4 and eLIFT scores (Appendix 1) are two simple blood tests for fibrosis that can be performed in clinical practice. The objective of this study was to assess primary care physicians' perception of chronic liver disease and their current practice regarding screening and management of these conditions.

POPULATION AND METHODS

This is a descriptive observational study of a cross-sectional nature among Family Medicine (FM) residents and primary care physicians (general practitioners and FM specialists) practicing in Tunisia. It was conducted from October 30, 2022 to February 10, 2023. It consisted in sending a questionnaire to physicians and residents specialized in Family Medicine in order to question them about their theoretical knowledge on chronic liver diseases, as well as their current practice concerning the screening and management of these pathologies. We sent the questionnaire to 148 members of the Tunisian Messenger group entitled "Family Medicine Specialists", and conducted a follow-up in a Tunisian facebook group entitled "Department of Family and Community Medicine" comprising 362 members.

Residents and physicians of other specialties as well as those not practicing in Tunisia were not included in this work. The questionnaire (Appendix 1) was written in the form of a Google Forms with 17 questions including 10 MCQs, 4 UQs, and 3 ROCQs. It was necessary to answer all the questions in order to validate participation. The response time was estimated at 10 minutes.

We conducted two succcssive reminders, each two months apart (October 30 and December 30) to increase the participation rate. Access to the questionnaire was closed on February 10, 2023.

We performed a descriptive analysis of the data using Excel software. The results are expressed as a percentage (%).

Participants were free to respond or not to the questionnaire and an introduction explaining the purpose of the study was attached online. Anonymity and confidentiality of data were assured.

RESULTS

I. CHARACTERISTICS OF THE STUDY POPULATION

Of the 42 physicians who responded to the questionnaire, 71% were women and 29% were men. The majority were family medicine residents (64%), between 26 and 30 years of age (67%), and practicing in an urban area (%). **Table 1** details the various characteristics of the study population.

Table 1: Characteristics of the study population

N		%
Gender		
Woman	30	71
Male	12	29
Age		
26-30	28	67
31-40	14	33
Grade		
Resident in Medicine of	27	64
Family		
Family Doctor	5	12
General Practitioner	10	24
Number of years in practice		
1-5	33	78
5-10	5	12
10-20	4	10
Zone geographical area		
exercise		
Rural	5	12
Semi-urban	5	12
Urban	32	76
Department of practice		
Hospital Center	26	62
university		
Regional Hospital	8	19
Basic health center	5	12
Private practice	3	7

II. THEORETICAL KNOWLEDGE OF PHYSICIANS GENERALISTS

The physicians surveyed underestimated the prevalence of chronic liver disease in their patients. Indeed, half of them (52.4%) thought that the prevalence of chronic liver disease in their patients was less than 5% (Figure 1).

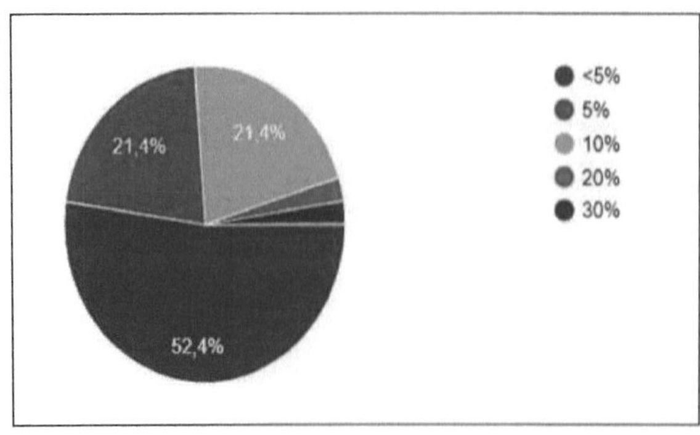

Figure 1: General practitioners' estimates of the prevalence of chronic liver disease in their patient population

The majority of them (80%) estimated that they had between 1 and 10% of their patients with cirrhosis (whether compensated or not) and underestimated the number of cirrhosis cases discovered at the decompensation stage, since **73.8%** thought that this represented only 20 to 40% of cases. **Only a quarter of** the respondents answered 60% (Figure 2)

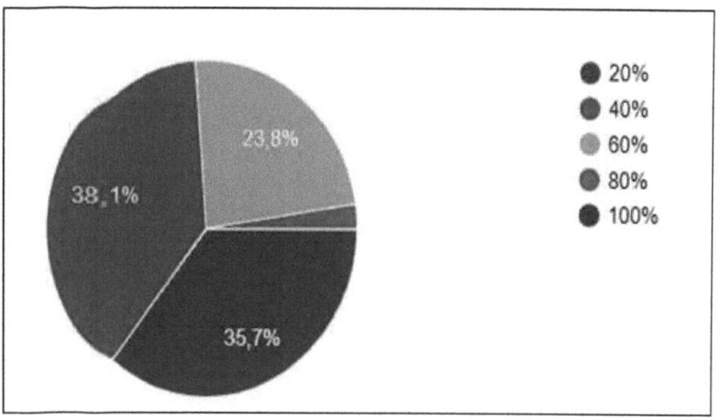

Figure 2: Estimated rate of cirrhosis revealed by a complication

The same is true for the rate of liver cancers diagnosed in the palliative stage; **21.4%** of physicians answered correctly 60% but **the majority** (73.8%) estimated this figure only between 20 and 40% of cases (Figure 3).

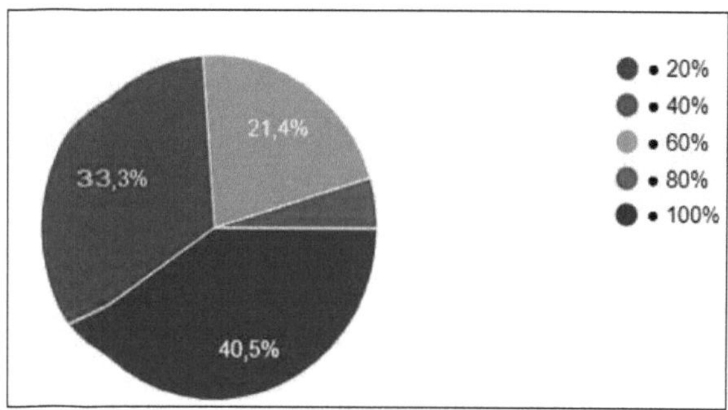

Figure 3: Estimated rate of primary liver cancers revealed at palliative stage

Regarding the etiologies of chronic liver disease, excessive alcohol consumption was cited as the primary cause by **54% of** physicians and hepatitis B by **36%**. However, **76%** agreed that the number of patients with hepatic steatosis had increased in their practice over the past 10 years. According to Table 2, the number of patients with viral hepatitis C or B was considered stable by **52%** and **50% of the** physicians respectively and decreasing for **less than half of them** (38% and 33%).

Table 2: Ranking of the five causes of chronic liver disease based on the study population

		n	%
Alcohol			
	Increase	23	55
	Stability	17	40
	Decrease	2	5
Chronic hepatitis B			
	Increase	7	17
	Stability	21	50
	Decrease	14	33
Chronic hepatitis C			
	Increase	4	10
	Stability	22	52
	Decrease	16	38
Hemochromatosis			
	Increase	6	14
	Stability	20	48
	Decrease	16	38
Non-alcoholic hepatic steatopathy			
	Increase	32	76
	Stability	7	17
	Decrease	3	7

Of the physicians interviewed in this study, 90.5% considered that they were not sufficiently informed about the management of chronic liver disease (Figure 5).

III. CURRENT PRACTICE OF GENERAL PRACTITIONERS

All of the physicians surveyed carried out regular monitoring of liver biology in their chronically ill patients. They instituted it in overweight or obese patients and in type 2 diabetic patients in 71.4% and **38.1% of cases** respectively.

This blood workup almost always included transaminases and GGT. Indeed, **97.6%** of physicians routinely measured AST and ALT and **90.5%** GGT. **Only 42.9%** of physicians included platelet counts. Only **66.7%** and **35.7%** of physicians prescribed PT and albumin determinations, respectively.

The majority of physicians performed this biological blood test every 6 months (**47.6%)** to one year (**47.6%**).

Regarding the main reasons for referring patients to a hepato-gastroenterologist, the majority of physicians cited the existence of a persistent disturbance of the liver biology. Indeed, **81%** referred patients when there was a persistent elevation of transaminases, and 73.8% when there was an elevation of GGT. Nearly half (45.2%) of the physicians said they referred their patients to the specialist when they showed signs of hepatic steatosis on liver ultrasound and 21.4% when there were risk factors for chronic liver disease, regardless of the results of complementary examinations. It should be noted that a minority of the physicians surveyed used the FIB4 (10%) and eLIFT (5%) fibrosis tests to guide their decision.

IV. USE OF NON-INVASIVE TESTS AND IMPLICATIONS

Of the physicians surveyed, **one-third (33.3%)** responded that they were familiar with non-invasive liver fibrosis tests.

Regarding the different tests they were aware of, **19%** of them mentioned FibroScan®, **10%** for FibroTest® and **10%** and **5%** respectively for the simple FIB4 and eLIFT tests.

After presentation of these last two simple tests, 57.1% of physicians responded that they would prefer to use the FIB4 in their daily practice over the eLIFT.

However, **16.7%** were not ready to use this type of test and considered that the hepato-gastroenterologist should assess the severity of chronic liver disease in all patients concerned. Using the example of the therapeutic management of chronic viral hepatitis C in the outpatient setting, **31%** of the physicians felt ready to treat their patients themselves and **11.9%** of them felt that it was also up to the hepato-gastroenterologist to manage the treatment. **47.6%** of them agreed to screen their patients with risk factors for HCV infection and **7.1% agreed to** screen all their patients systematically.

DISCUSSION

I. DISCUSSION GENERAL

General practitioners have an important role to play in the early detection of chronic liver diseases. The challenge is to recognize and target at an early stage the patients to be referred to the hepato-gastroenterologist for an adapted management.

1. Theoretical knowledge of general practitioners

In our study, a lack of information concerning all chronic liver diseases was recognized by 90.5% of general practitioners. They clearly underestimated the prevalence of these diseases and their complications. On the other hand, they overestimate the rate of cirrhosis ("compensated" or not) in their patients. Due to a lack of knowledge, they may confuse cirrhosis with chronic liver disease.

Non-alcoholic fatty liver disease (NAFLD) has become a major cause of liver disease worldwide (4). In our study, 76% of physicians see it in their daily practice. The global prevalence of NAFLD is 25.24%

(95% CI: 22.10-28.65), with the highest prevalence in the Middle East and South America and the lowest in Africa (4).

Chronic alcoholism remains the leading etiology responsible for cirrhosis and primary liver cancer (6) and is the second leading cause of chronic liver disease after NAFLD (3). Nevertheless, in our study, alcohol was still cited by half of the physicians surveyed as the primary cause of liver disease. Moreover, 55% of the physicians note an increase in the number of their patients with excessive alcohol consumption over the last 10 years. This finding may be related to the fact that the issue of alcohol consumption is being discussed more systematically in consultations.The prevalence of hepatitis C, according to the Tunisian national survey data was 0.87% in the general population. The national prevalence of HBsAg was also low, estimated at 1.7% according to a population-based study, thus classifying Tunisia as a low endemic countries (14). Furthermore, the number of patients with viral hepatitis C or B was considered stable by physicians at 52% and 50% respectively and decreasing for less than half of them (38% and 33%).

2. CURRENT PRACTICE OF GENERAL PRACTITIONERS

2.1.Carrying out of the hepatic function assessment

In our study, all general practitioners declared that they regularly monitored the liver biology of their chronically ill patients (every 6 months to one year). On the other hand, only 38.1% of them prescribe it for their type 2 diabetic patients, probably because they associate this pathology less with the risk of developing chronic liver disease. However, it is necessary to identify the main risk factors for the development of NAFLD, namely insulin resistance, overweight, obesity, type 2 diabetes and metabolic syndrome. Indeed, in some patients, simple hepatic steatosis can progress to non-alcoholic steatohepatitis (NASH), which can sometimes lead to liver cirrhosis and its complications, including hepatocellular carcinoma (15) . It is imperative to screen these patients in primary care so that they can be managed by a hepatogastroenterologist. Indeed, according to the American Association for the Study of Liver Disease guidelines, there should be systematic screening for NAFLD, at least in high-risk individuals with diabetes or obesity (16).

The complete hepatic biologic workup, including AST, ALT, GGT, alkaline phosphatases, platelets, PT, bilirubin and albumin, is rarely performed in the practice of general practitioners, but the majority of physicians perform at least transaminases (97.6%) and GGT (90.5%). This could be explained by the fact that two thirds of the physicians interviewed are not aware of non-invasive tests for liver fibrosis, and therefore are not aware of the usefulness of other biological parameters.

2.2. Referral to specialist

The majority of patients are referred to the hepato-gastroenterologist for a blood test, probably because it is a more easily and quickly accessible complementary test than liver ultrasound in primary care. Thus, it is possible that general practitioners are content to refer their patients to the specialist. However, liver ultrasound is not necessary to assess a patient's risk of fibrosis using non-invasive tests, but these are still not well known (17).

Moreover, our study shows that 21.4% of practitioners refer patients with risk factors to the hepato-gastroenterologist, regardless of the results of complementary examinations, and almost half (45.2%) do so when the patient has hepatic steatosis found on ultrasound. This practice is responsible for many "futile" specialist consultations since the management of simple steatosis, i.e. without evidence of advanced fibrosis, is based on the introduction of hygienic and dietary measures and the control of risk factors (16).

2.3.Use of tests of screening and future involvement

2.3.1. Use of non-invasive fibrosis tests in primary care

Non-invasive tests for liver fibrosis are not known by the majority of physicians surveyed. Indeed, only one third of them claim to be aware of them. FibroScan® is the most cited, by 19% of them. This is an elastometry device which, using a probe placed on the skin, measures the hardness of the liver, which is directly related to the degree of hepatic fibrosis. Its use is quick and painless (12). The availability of these devices in the public sector is still low in Tunisia.

Blood tests such as the FibroMeter® and FibroTest® are less familiar to primary care practitioners. They use more specialized blood parameters and are more accurate than simple blood tests in assessing liver fibrosis (12).

In order to allow early detection of liver fibrosis by the general practitioner and to target patients requiring further investigations and a specialized hepatology consultation, simple and reliable blood tests have been developed, notably: the eLIFT and FIB4 scores (17).

These tests are still largely unknown, since few physicians cited FIB4 (10%) and eLIFT (5%). Nevertheless, 83.3% of the physicians surveyed would be willing to use them in their daily practice to assess the risk of fibrosis in their patients with risk factors. There is therefore a real interest in informing primary care physicians about the existence of new tools that can optimize the patient's pathway.

In their daily practice, more than half of the physicians (57.1%) would choose to use the FIB4. We can assume that they prefer it to eLIFT because PT is a parameter of the latter, and it is often forgotten when prescribing a blood liver test in daily practice. This could lead to a limitation in its use, especially by physicians who would not want to call their patients for consultation several times.

2.3.2. Investment of general practitioners in the management of chronic viral hepatitis C

The current treatment of chronic viral hepatitis C has undergone a real boom since the appearance of the new direct antivirals. These treatments have produced better results than previous treatments, with sustained virological responses often exceeding 90%. Treatment regimens have also been considerably simplified since the development of new molecules active on all HCV genotypes. These pangenotypic treatments have made it possible to create a simplified care pathway and thus open the way to management by general practitioners for patients not at risk. This strategy, aimed at universal treatment of hepatitis C cases, has been adopted by several countries. In Tunisia, on the other hand, since pangenotypic antivirals are still not available, combination treatments consisting of two or three molecules are currently indicated and prescribed exclusively by hepatologists and infectiologists.In our study, while waiting for the availability of pangenotypic combinations, less than half of the physicians felt ready to treat those eligible for simplified treatment themselves. This may be related to a lack of communication regarding the management modalities in primary care, hence the importance of updating the information.Only 47.6% of physicians plan to screen patients at risk for HCV, while it is recommended that all patients be screened for hepatitis C. person at risk of HCV infection or who believes that he or she may have had contact with HCV HCV, or for which the health care provider believes there is a risk (10).

II. STRENGTHS AND LIMITATIONS OF THE STUDY

1. POINT STRONG

The strong point of our work is its originality since it is the first study in Tunisia evaluating the practices of primary care physicians and their pedagogical learning needs concerning the management of chronic liver diseases.

2. L IMITES

▶ The use of a self-administered questionnaire could be a limitation in our study. Without the investigator to conduct the questionnaire, respondents could encounter difficulties in understanding the questions.

▶ The sample is relatively small and heterogeneous. Further, more focused studies should include all family medicine residents from different medical schools

▶ It is possible that the writing of certain questions in the form of MCQs may have led to a confusion bias, particularly those concerning the management carried out by doctors. For example, we assume that the rate of prescription of certain parameters of the biological blood test such as PT or albumin was overestimated and that fewer general practitioners perform these tests in routine practice than is reflected in the results of our study. The choice of proposals may have influenced the respondents to tick them.

CONCLUSION

The results of our study reveal an under-perception of chronic liver diseases by general practitioners. Indeed, they underestimate the prevalence and impact of these diseases, and do not screen them in an optimal manner since they do not systematically target all populations at risk. In addition, the biological blood tests that they perform in routine practice rarely include all the parameters necessary for a complete evaluation of liver function.

Practitioners believe that this lack of appreciation of chronic liver disease is attributed to a lack of information, but they are willing to be trained and to modify their practices. In order to allow targeted screening and appropriate referral of patients in the health care system, it is important that general practitioners be aware of the existence of accessible, simple and rapid tools such as the eLIFT or FIB4 scores and integrate them into their consultations. Thus, an earlier diagnosis of liver fibrosis would make it possible to offer curative treatment to patients, before the stages of decompensated cirrhosis or palliative liver cancer, in particular with new drugs that should soon be available for the management of NAFLD.

However, general practitioners do not consider treating patients with chronic viral hepatitis C themselves. Information and training of primary care physicians, especially family medicine residents, is therefore essential so that they can actively participate in the therapeutic management of these patients.

In conclusion, the presentation of hepatic fibrosis screening tools and recommendations could be integrated into the continuing education of primary care physicians, through presentations by hepatologists at conferences or training days in order to standardize practices.

REFERENCES

1. Vogel A, Meyer T, Sapisochin G, Salem R, Saborowski A. Hepatocellular carcinoma. Lancet Lond Engl. 15 Oct 2022;400(10360):1345-62.

2. Ginès P, Krag A, Abraldes JG, Solà E, Fabrellas N, Kamath PS. Liver cirrhosis. Lancet Lond Engl. 9 Oct 2021;398(10308):1359-76.

3. NASH (EASL-2017 recommendations) [Internet]. FMC-HGE. [cited March 4, 2023]. Available from: https://www.fmcgastro.org/texte-postu/postu-2019-paris/nash-recommendations-easl-2017/

4. Younossi ZM, Koenig AB, Abdelatif D, Fazel Y, Henry L, Wymer M. Global epidemiology of nonalcoholic fatty liver disease-Meta-analytic assessment of prevalence, incidence, and outcomes. Hepatol Baltim Md. Jul 2016;64(1):73-84.

5. Grattagliano I, D'Ambrosio G, Palmieri VO, Moschetta A, Palasciano G, Portincasa P, et al. Improving nonalcoholic fatty liver disease management by general practitioners: a critical evaluation and impact of an educational training program. J Gastrointest Liver Dis JGLD. Dec 2008;17(4):389-94.

6. Alcoholic liver disease (EASL-2018 recommendations) [Internet]. FMC-HGE. [cited March 4, 2023]. Available from: https://www.fmcgastro.org/texte-postu/postu-2019- paris/alcoholic-liver-disease-recommendations-easl-2018/.

7. Alcoholism widespread among Tunisians: Causes, effects and treatments (Addictologist) [Internet]. Gnet news. 2022 [cited 17 Feb 2023]. Available from: https://news.gnet.tn/alcoolisme/

8. Nguyen MH, Wong G, Gane E, Kao JH, Dusheiko G. Hepatitis B Virus: Advances in Prevention, Diagnosis, and Therapy. Clin Microbiol Rev. March 18, 2020;33(2):e00046- 19.

9. D'Amico G, Garcia-Tsao G, Pagliaro L. Natural history and prognostic indicators of survival in cirrhosis: a systematic review of 118 studies. J Hepatol. Jan 2006;44(1):217-31.

10. Hepatitis C: simplified management in adults [Internet]. Haute Autorité de Santé. [cited March 12, 2023]. Available from: https://www.has- sante.fr/jcms/c_2911891/en/hepatitis-c-simplified-management-in-adults

11. JFHOD | SNFGE.org - French medical society of hepato-gastroenterology and digestive oncology digestive oncology [Internet]. [cited 12 March 2023]. Available at:

https://www.snfge.org/content/le-easy-liver-fibrosis-test-elift-permet-deviter-des- evaluations-non-invasive-of-fibrosis

12. Non-invasive methods [Internet]. AFEF - French Society of Hepatology. [cited 10 March 2023]. Available At: https://afef.asso.fr/la-maladie/les-examens- specifics/noninvasive-methods/

13. walid. The prevalence rate of hepatitis B in Tunisia | Directinfo [Internet]. 2013 [cited 4 March 2023]. Available at: https://directinfo.webmanagercenter.com/2013/10/26/le-taux-de-prevalence-de- lhepatitis-b-in-tunisia-between-4-and-7/

14. Ben Hadj Boudali M, Hazgui O, Bouguerra H, Saffar F, Hannachi N, Bahri O, et al. Hepatitis B in Tunisia. Epidemiology, risk factors and impact of vaccination. Rev Epidemiology Public Health. May 1, 2019;67:S158.

15. Juanola O, Martínez-López S, Francés R, Gómez-Hurtado I. Non-Alcoholic Fatty Liver Disease: Metabolic, Genetic, Epigenetic and Environmental Risk Factors. Int J Environ Res Public Health. 14 May 2021;18(10):5227.

16. Chalasani N, Younossi Z, Lavine JE, Charlton M, Cusi K, Rinella M, et al. The diagnosis and management of nonalcoholic fatty liver disease: practice guidance from the American Association for the Study of Liver Diseases. Hepatology. jan 2018;67(1):328.

17. Loomba R, Adams LA. Advances in non-invasive assessment of hepatic fibrosis. Gut. Jul 2020;69(7):1343-52.

APPENDIX

PRIMARY CARE PHYSICIAN QUESTIONNAIRE

Chronic liver diseases can progress to cirrhosis and liver cancer. New, highly effective treatments are now available and more will become available in the near future.

As part of our thesis work in general practice, we are asking you to answer a questionnaire of 17 MCQs in order to evaluate the perception of chronic liver diseases in primary care.

Completing this questionnaire will take no more than 10 minutes. We thank you in advance for your participation.

ABOUT YOU

A. You are :

- A woman
- A man

B. In which structure do you work?

- In the office, alone
- In a group practice
- Multidisciplinary health center
- Other (specify):

C. In which geographical area do you practice?

- Rural
- Semi-urban
- Urban

D. In which department do you practice?

E. What is your year of birth?

F. How long have you been practicing medicine?

- Less than 5 years
- 5 to 10 years
- 10 to 20 years
- 20 to 30 years
- Over 30 years old

QUESTIONNAIRE

1) What is your estimate of the prevalence of chronic liver disease in your patient population?

- <5%
- 5%
- 10%
- 20%
- 30%

2) Chronic liver disease can progress to cirrhosis. Initially, cirrhosis is said to be "compensated", and then complications arise ("decompensated cirrhosis" with ascites, jaundice, hepatic encephalopathy, digestive haemorrhage due to rupture of an oesophageal varicose vein, or hepatocellular carcinoma). In your opinion, what is the rate of cirrhosis revealed by a complication, i.e., the rate of cirrhosis diagnosed at the decompensation stage?

- 20%
- 40%
- 60%
- 80%
- 100%

3) How many cirrhotic patients (compensated and decompensated) do you estimate are in your patient population (indicate a number from 0 to 100%)?

4) Primary liver cancers (hepatocellular carcinoma) that are not very advanced can be treated curatively (surgery, radiofrequency, liver transplantation), while more advanced cancers can only be treated palliatively (chemo-embolization, chemotherapy, radiotherapy). In your opinion, what is the rate of hepatocellular carcinomas diagnosed too late, i.e. diagnosed at the palliative stage?

- 20%
- 40%
- 60%
- 80%
- 100%

5) Among the following situations, please indicate for which of the following you initiate a follow-up regular liver biology (check the corresponding box(es))?

- Chronic ethylism
- Asthenia
- Type 2 diabetes

- Overweight/obesity
- Cardiovascular diseases

6) For this regular liver monitoring, what do you include in your check-up liver biology (check the corresponding box(es))?

- ASAT
- ALAT
- Gamma-GT
- Alkaline phosphatases
- Bilirubin
- Plates
- TP
- Albumin

7) How often do you perform this liver biology monitoring?

- Every 3 months
- Every 6 months
- Every year
- Every 2 years
- Every 3 years

8) In your current practice, on what grounds do you decide to refer a patient to a specialized hepato-gastroenterology consultation (check

the corresponding box(es))?

- As soon as there is a risk factor (excessive alcohol consumption, obesity...) whatever the results of the complementary examinations (biological liver tests, ultrasound...)
- Hepatic steatosis on liver ultrasound
- Persistent elevation of gamma-GT
- Persistent elevation of transaminases
- Persistent elevation of ferritin levels
- Other (specify):

9) What is the rate of patients with liver abnormalities (biology, ultrasound) that you estimate to be referred to the hepato-gastroenterologist in your practice (indicate a figure from 0 to 100%)?

10) Do you know about non-invasive liver fibrosis tests?

- No
- Yes

11) If yes, which ones (free response)?

12) Non-invasive fibrosis tests are used to assess the degree of hepatic fibrosis in chronic liver diseases. Their interest is therefore to identify early patients who develop an advanced form of liver disease while they are still asymptomatic. Here are two fibrosis blood tests, simple to perform in clinical practice: the FIB4 and the eLIFT.

<table>
<tr>
<td>The eLIFT is calculated by hand, without the need for a calculator, using points assigned to each variable.
<table>
<tr><th>eLIFT</th><th></th><th>POINTS</th></tr>
<tr><td>Age ≥40 ans</td><td></td><td>3</td></tr>
<tr><td>Sexe masculin</td><td></td><td>1</td></tr>
<tr><td>ASAT (UI/L)</td><td>• 35 - 69
• ≥70</td><td>2
4</td></tr>
<tr><td>GGT (UI/L)</td><td>• 35 - 89
• ≥90</td><td>1
2</td></tr>
<tr><td>Plaquettes (G/L)</td><td>• 170 - 249
• <170</td><td>1
4</td></tr>
<tr><td>TP (%)</td><td>• 84 - 96
• <84</td><td>2
4</td></tr>
</table>
</td>
<td>The FIB4 requires a computer calculation:

$$FIB4 = \frac{\text{Age (années) x ASAT (UI/l)}}{\text{Plaquettes (G/l) x } \sqrt{\text{ALAT (UI/l)}}}$$

Free calculators are available on the web (example https://www.hepatitisc.uw.edu/page/clinical- calculators/fib-4).</td>
</tr>
<tr>
<td>A result of 2:8 indicates a risk of advanced hepatic fibrosis with the need for explorations specialized.</td>
<td>A result of 2:1.30 indicates a risk of advanced hepatic fibrosis with the need for specialized explorations.</td>
</tr>
</table>

Which of these two non-invasive fibrosis tests would you prefer to use in your clinical practice?

- FIB4
- eLIFT

13) Would you be willing to use this type of test to assess the severity of liver damage in your alcoholic or obese patients?

- Yes, and depending on the result I will decide to refer the patient to the hepato-gastroenterologist
- No, it is up to the hepato-gastroenterologist to assess the severity of chronic liver disease at all patients concerned

14) Rank these causes of chronic liver disease from 1 to 5, according to your opinion of the most frequent (number 1) to the least frequent (number 5) :

- Alcohol:
- Chronic hepatitis B:
- Chronic hepatitis C:
- Hemochromatosis:
- Non-alcoholic fatty liver disease (NAFLD/NASH):

15) In your patient base, what changes have you seen in these five causes of chronic liver disease over the past 10 years? For each proposition, grade: A (increase), S (stability), or D (decrease)?

- Alcohol:
- Chronic hepatitis B:
- Chronic hepatitis C:
- Hemochromatosis:
- Non-alcoholic fatty liver disease (NAFLD/NASH):

16) You feel sufficiently informed about the latest new products regarding the management of chronic liver diseases?

- Yes
- No

17) Since 2019, management of chronic hepatitis C has been greatly simplified with highly effective treatments (one pill per day, 12 weeks of treatment, very few side effects, and >95% cure rate). Antiviral treatment can now be prescribed by general practitioners if specialized fibrosis blood tests (FibroMeter®, FibroTest®) indicate the absence of severe liver fibrosis. Will this change your practices (check the corresponding box(es))?

- No, I will not change my current practice
- No, the management of chronic hepatitis C is a matter for hepato-gastroenterologists
- Yes, I will now screen my patients for chronic hepatitis C (prescribe serology), routinely for all patients
- Yes, I will now screen my patients for chronic hepatitis C (prescription of serology), but only in patients with risk factors (history of transfusion, IV drug use, etc.)
- Yes, and within the framework of the new recommendations I am considering treating patients with chronic hepatitis C myself

SUMMARY

Assessment of the perception of chronic liver disease by primary care physicians in Tunisia

Introduction: Chronic liver diseases can progress to cirrhosis and liver cancer. Because of their long silent progression, their diagnosis is still too late. New highly effective treatments are now available and others will become available very soon. The objective of this study was to evaluate the perception of chronic liver diseases by primary care physicians, as well as their current practice regarding the screening and management of these pathologies.

Subjects and methods: This is an observational, cross-sectional study, conducted from October 30, 2022 to February 10, 2023, which consisted of sending a questionnaire to residents and primary care physicians practicing in Tunisia.

Results: Of the 42 physicians who responded to the questionnaire, 71% were women and 29% were men; 64% were family medicine residents. The majority of the 42 responding physicians underestimated the prevalence of chronic liver disease and its complications. Regular monitoring of liver biology was performed by the physicians surveyed in all alcohol-dependent patients, 71.4% of obese patients and 38.1% of type 2 diabetics. This biological blood test almost always included transaminases and GGT, whereas PT and albumin were only prescribed by 66.7% and 35.7% of physicians respectively. One third of the physicians (33.3%) responded that they were aware of non-invasive liver fibrosis tests. Nevertheless, they would be generally willing to use these tests in their daily practice. On the other hand, although simplified treatment could be accessible in primary care, they do not wish to treat patients with chronic viral hepatitis C themselves.

Conclusion: Primary care physicians have expressed a willingness to be trained and to change their practice, particularly through the use of simple blood tests for advanced fibrosis. This would allow earlier diagnosis of liver fibrosis and offer curative treatment of chronic liver disease before the advanced stages of cirrhosis and hepatocellular carcinoma.

Keywords: chronic liver disease, primary care physicians, blood tests simple

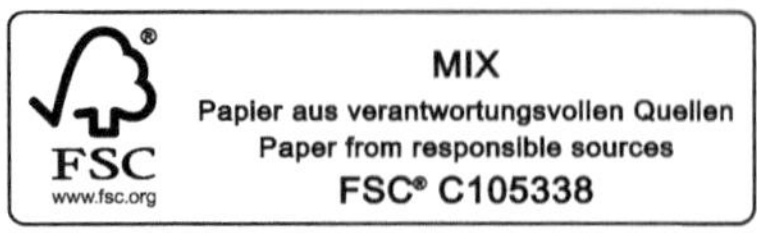

Printed by Books on Demand GmbH, Norderstedt / Germany